Nursing Pocket Guide

Deborah Antai-Otong,
MS, APRN, BC, FAAN
Continuous Readiness Officer
Program Manager
Care Coordination Home Telehealth
Psychiatric Mental Health
Nurse Practitioner
Veterans Integrated Services
Network, (VISN) 17
Arlington, Texas

JONES AND BARTLETT PUBLISHERS
Sudbury, Massachusetts
BOSTON   TORONTO   LONDON   SINGAPORE

World Headquarters

Jones and Bartlett Publishers
40 Tall Pine Drive
Sudbury, MA 01776
978-443-5000
info@jbpub.com
www.jbpub.com

Jones and Bartlett Publishers
Canada
6339 Ormindale Way
Mississauga, Ontario L5V 1J2
Canada

Jones and Bartlett Publishers
International
Barb House, Barb Mews
London W6 7PA
United Kingdom

Copyright © 2009 by Jones and Bartlett Publishers, LLC
ISBN: 978-0-7637-5413-6

Production Credits
Executive Editor: Kevin Sullivan
Acquisitions Editor: Emily Ekle
Acquisitions Editor: Amy Sibley
Editorial Assistant: Patricia Donnelly
Production Director: Amy Rose
Production Editor: Carolyn F. Rogers
Associate Marketing Manager: Ilana Goddess
Manufacturing Buyer: Amy Bacus
Composition: Graphic World
Text Design: Anne Spencer
Cover Design: Kristin E. Ohlin
Printing and Binding: Imago
Cover Printing: Imago

6048

Printed in China
12 11 10 09 08   10 9 8 7 6 5 4 3 2 1

Contents

- Section 1: Introduction   1
- Section 2: Normal Neuroanatomy and Physiology   5
- Section 3: Assessment   19
- Section 4: Specific Psychiatric Disorders   33
- Section 5: Pharmacological and Psychotherapeutic Interventions   55
- Section 6: Legal and Ethical Considerations   79
- Section 7: Psychiatric Emergencies   85
- Section 8: Psychotherapeutic Approaches   99

and provision of care have become an integral aspect of psychiatric services (Richmond, Hollander, Ackerson, Robinson, Gracias, Shults, et al.; 2007). Chief advantages of emergency mental health services include expediting access to treatment of the client with a psychiatric disorder, ensuring client and staff safety, thwarting a crisis or decreasing its potential deleterious effects, and synthesizing data to make an accurate diagnosis and appropriate disposition. The purpose of this book is to provide a guide for nurses in psychiatric and diverse practice settings to assess, evaluate, and treat clients who present with psychiatric disorders across the life span. This book is divided into several sections that provide a strong foundation for psychiatric diagnosis, treatment management, and appropriate disposition. It also provides guiding principles of psychiatric care followed by a brief overview of neuroanatomy and target sites for pharmacological and psychotherapeutic interventions.

▉ Guiding Principles of Psychiatric Care (Assessment)

Data collection, evaluation, and diagnosis require a systematic process based on theoretical framework, practice guidelines, and evidence-based practice. The underpinnings of psychiatric conditions are multidimensional and complex and stem from neurobiological, genetic, cultural, psychosocial, socioeconomic, and environmental factors that underscore adaptive and maladaptive responses across the life span. Emerging data implicate the role of prenatal and early postnatal factors that determine one's capacity to develop and maintain meaningful relationships, tolerate stress, manage anxiety effectively, and adapt to change. Psychiatric disorders are brain disorders, and the upcoming sections provide a synopsis of major brain regions and function. Neuroimaging findings have elucidated specific brain regions associated with psychiatric disorders and provide a wealth of data important to clinicians and their clients concerning treatment options. Understanding these multidimensional processes creates a foundation for linking target brain regions to specific psychiatric symptoms, treatment approaches, and positive clinical outcomes. Section 2 provides a brief synopsis of specific brain regions and target sites for pharmacological interventions.

Reference

Richmond, T. S., Hollander, J. E., Ackerson, T. H., Robinson, K., Gracias, V., Shults, J., et al. (2007). Psychiatric disorders in patients presenting to the Emergency Department for minor injury. *Nursing Research, 56,* 275–282.

B. Brain (**Figure 2-2**)
- Cerebrum: anterior or upper and largest part of the brain
  Cerebral cortex is the surface of the cerebrum that is divided into four major lobes (Pierri & Lewis, 2005):
  - Frontal: involved in executive function, such as reasoning, ability to abstract, calculation, planning, judgment, parts of speech and movement, and ascribing meaning and emotional relevance to events
  - Parietal: involved in movement, recognition, perception of stimuli, orientation
  - Temporal: involved in perceptions, recognition of auditory stimuli, memory and speech, and taste
  - Occipital: associated with visual processing
- Cerebellum: portion of the brain consisting of two hemispheres located behind and above the medulla; coordinates motor activities and maintains body equilibrium
- Brainstem: annexes the hemispheres of the brain, cerebellum, and spinal cord; responsible for vital life function (e.g., breathing, heart beat, blood pressure)
  - Midbrain: involved in vision, hearing, eye movement, and body movement
  - Medulla: involved in life function, heart beat, breathing
  - Pons: involved in motor control and sensory analysis

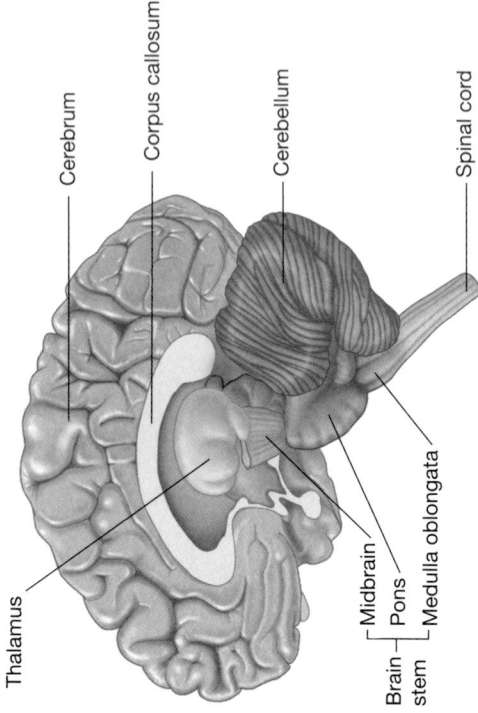

Figure 2-2   Neuroanatomical structures of the brain.

- Corpus callosum: connects the two cerebral hemispheres and is essential in the coordination of activities between the hemispheres, particularly when specific tasks are limited to one hemisphere
- Reticular formation: critical for maintaining wakefulness and referred to as the reticular activating system

1. Neuroanatomical Structures
   - Amygdala: Located in the medial temporal lobe. Implicated in fear responses and pathogenesis of anxiety disorders.
   - Prefrontal cortex: Part of the cerebrum responsible for goal-directed behavior, ability to concentrate, and short-term and recall memory. It exerts inhibitory influence over the limbic system and physiological areas of the cerebrum. It is implicated in the perception of ascription of meaning to an event. It regulates emotional and fear responses and interfaces with the hippocampus and amygdala to ascribe relevance and significance of external stimuli and is believed to play a role in the pathogenesis of anxiety disorders, such as posttraumatic stress disorder and obsessive-compulsive disorder (Pierri & Lewis, 2005).
   - Limbic system: Buried within the cerebrum and often referred to as the "emotional brain." It is the neural substrate for emotional experience and expression, and it includes other structures,

such as the hypothalamus, amygdala, thalamus, and hippocampus, involved in the modulation of emotions (Rauch, Shin, & Phelps, 2006).

- Hippocampus: Located in temporal lobe and forms part of the limbic system and plays a role in memory and spatial navigation. It is involved in the processing and transfer of information into memory and memory consolidation.
- Basal ganglia system: Mass of nuclei that play a pivotal role in modulating movement and cognitive function.
- Hypothalamus: Small structure that is a critical part of the neural circuitry involved in the modulation of emotions, autonomic nervous system activity, temperature regulation, feeding responses, and endocrine and physiological functions. It interfaces with limbic system, brainstem, and spinal cord and regulates the pituitary gland function. It is important for learning and memory, converting short-term and permanent memory, memory recall, and spatial relationships in the world.
- Thalamus: Located medial to the basal ganglia and serves as the chief synaptic relay station for information reaching the cerebral cortex.

2. Neurocircuitry and Nerve Impulse
   - Neurons: Electrically excitable cells in the nervous system that process and transmit information. They communicate via chemical and electrical

  synapses in a process referred to as
  synaptic transmission.
- Synapse: The area in which a nerve impulse transmits from an axon on one
  neuron to the dendrite of another by
  chemical and electrical conduction.
  Synapses at distinct sites use different
  neurotransmitters.
  - Presynaptic neuron: toward the
    synapse
  - Postsynaptic neuron: away from the
    synapse
3. Neurotransmitter
- Chemical product of the nervous system
  that makes possible the movement of the
  nerve impulse across the synapse
  (Paterson, Trachtenberg, Thompson,
  Belliveau, & Beggs, 2006); most have
  more than one function (**Table 2-1**)
4. Neuroendocrine System
- Hypothalamus-pituitary-adrenal (HPA):
  A major part of the neuroendocrine
  system that modulates reactions to
  stress. It is the mechanism for activating interactions among glands, hor-
  mones, and parts of the midbrain that
  activates adaptive biological and behavioral coping responses.
  Dysregulation of this axis is implicated
  in the pathogenesis of chronic stress
  responses and some anxiety disorders,
  such as posttraumatic stress disorder
  (Antai-Otong, 2007; Rauch, Shin, &
  Phelps, 2006).
5. Cranial nerve function (**Table 2-2**)

Table 2-1   Major Neurotransmitters: Target Sites for Psychopharmacological Agents

Substance	Effect	Function	Clinical Example/Target Sites for Medications
Acetylcholine	Excitatory or inhibitory	Memory	Alzheimer's disease associated with reduced acetylcholine-producing neurons
			Target site for anticholinesterase medications
Monoamines			
Dopamine	Excitatory	Memory, cognition, attention, motor activity, motivation, please and reward system, regulation of prolactin, sleep, mood, attention, and learning	Schizophrenia and other psychotic disorders associated with increased or dysregulation
			Parkinson's disease associated with destruction of dopamine-producing neurons
			Decreased levels associated with movement disorders, including extrapyramidal symptoms, tardive dyskinesia
			Plays a role in attention deficit hyperactivity disorder
			Target site for antipsychotic medications

continues

Norepinephrine	Excitatory or inhibitory	Attention and focus "Fight-or-flight" stress response	Decreased levels associated with depression; increased levels associated with anxiety disorders Target site for antianxiety and antidepressant medications
Serotonin	Inhibitory	Plays crucial role in sleep, appetite, mood, impulsivity, and suicide risk	Decreased levels associated with depression, anxiety, appetite, and sleep disorders Serotonergic system affected in the brain and in peripheral immune cells of depressed patients Target site for antidepressant and antianxiety medications Alterations in multiple medullary serotonergic systems may contribute to the pathogenesis of sudden infant death
Amino Acids Gamma-aminobutyric acid	Inhibitory	Produce calming effects and are target sites for benzodiazepines	Decreased levels associated with anxiety disorders Target site for antianxiety and anticonvulsant medications

Table 2-1 Major Neurotransmitters: Target Sites for Psychopharmacological Agents, continued

Substance	Effect	Function	Clinical Example/Target Sites for Medications
Glutamate, aspartate	Excitatory	Involved in learning and memory	Alterations in production may play a role in the underpinnings of neurodegenerative disorders, such as Alzheimer's disease and schizophrenia
Glycine	Inhibitory	When released in synapse makes postsynaptic membrane more permeable to CL− and hyperpolarizes the membrane, making it less likely to polarize	Glycine found in the spinal cord and forebrain but precise role in the forebrain unclear
Neuropeptides			
Endorphins and enkephalins	Inhibitory	Most common neurotransmitters in the hypothalamus Inhibits firing of locus coeruleus	Low levels are associated with anxiety disorders Pain reduction associated with binding with narcotics on presynaptic neurons that block the release of these neurotransmitters
Substance P	Excitatory	Located in the pain transmission pathways	Increased levels found in chronic methamphetamine exposure Blocking its release with a narcotic reduces pain

Table 2-2 Cranial Nerves and Assessment Guide

Cranial Nerve	How Assessed
I: Olfactory	Ask client to close eyes and occlude one nostril and sniff a nonirritating substance, such as cloves, vanilla, or coffee. Ask to identify specific odors. Test each nostril separately.
II: Optic	Use Snellen eye chart to evaluate vision and visual field. Initially ask if client sees finger; move into visual fields. Use ophthalmoscope to assess blood vessels of interior eye.
III: Oculomotor	Assess pupils for shape, symmetry, and papillary reflex using a pen light; ability to follow moving objects.
IV: Trochlear	Tested concurrently with cranial nerve III involving ability to follow objects.
V: Trigeminal	Test sensations of pain, touch, and temperature with safety pin; hot and cold objects; test corneal reflex with cotton wisp, test motor branch by asking client to clench teeth, open mouth against resistance, and move jaw side to side. Allows clinician to detect deviation of jaw or asymmetry of muscle contraction.
VI: Abducens	Test concurrently with cranial nerve III associated with ability to move each eye laterally. Damage to nerve is evidenced by decreased ability to abduct the eye.

continues

Table 2-2   Cranial Nerves and Assessment Guide, continued

Cranial Nerve	How Assessed
VII: Facial	Assess two-thirds of tongue for ability to taste sweet, salty, sour, and bitter substances. Check facial symmetry; ask client to close eyes, smile, whistle, raise eyebrows, wrinkle forehead, etc. Assess tearing with ammonia fumes.
VIII: Vestibulocochlear (acoustic)	Test gross hearing by using air and bone conduction by using a tuning fork.
IX: Glossopharyngeal	Assess gag and swallowing reflexes. Ask client to speak and cough. Assess posterior one-third of tongue for taste.
X: Vagus	Test is the same as cranial nerve IX.
XI: Spinal Accessory	Assess sternocleidomastoid and trapezius muscles by asking client to rotate head and shrug shoulders against resistance. Observe for drooping or displacement of scapula.
XII: Hypoglossal	Ask client to stick out tongue and move tongue in all directions and subsequent position abnormalities assessed.

References

Antai-Otong, D. (2007). Unforgettable: Responding to PTSD in primary care. *Advance for Nurse Practitioners, 15,* 71–74.

Frankel, P. S., Alburges, M. E., Bush, L., Hanson, G. R., & Kish, S. J. (2007). Brain levels of neuropeptides in human chronic methamphetamine users. *Neuropharmacology, 53,* 447–454.

Paterson, D. S., Trachtenberg, F. L., Thompson, E. G., Belliveau, R. A., Beggs, A. H., & Darnall, R. (2006). Multiple serotonergic brainstem abnormalities in sudden infant death syndrome. *Journal of the American Medical Association, 296,* 2124–2132.

Pierri, J. N., & Lewis, D. A. (2005). Functional neuroanatomy. In B. J. Sadock & V. A. Sadock (Eds.), *Kaplan & Sadock's comprehensive textbook of psychiatry* (8th ed., pp. 3–32). Philadelphia: Lippincott Williams & Wilkins.

Rauch, S., Shin, L. M., & Phelps, E. A. (2006). Neurocircuitry models of post traumatic stress disorder and extinctions: Past, present and future. *Biological Psychiatry, 60,* 376–382.

Sadock, B. J., Sadock, V. A., & Sussman, N. (2006). *Kaplan & Sadock's pocket handbook of psychiatric drug treatment* (4th ed.). Philadelphia: Lippincott Williams & Wilkins.

B. Diagnostic and Laboratory Studies
- Chemistry profile
- Liver and renal function panels
- Electrolytes
- Complete blood count with differential
- Hematocrit and hemoglobin
- Thiamine, vitamin B_{12}, and folate levels
- Thyroid panel
- Comprehensive metabolic profile
- Pregnancy test (childbearing age group)
- Blood and urine cultures
- Toxicology screens
- Magnetic resonance imaging
- Electrocardiogram
- Chest x-ray

C. Physical Examination
- Vital signs
- Focused review of systems
- Review of cranial nerve (when indicated)
- Neurological signs
- Signs of head injury
- Eyes: pupil size, reaction to light, nystagmus
- Abnormal movements, hyperreflexia, gait
- Neck rigidity
- Breath for unusual odor

D. Mental Status Examination
  1. General description
  - Appearance: hygiene, grooming, etc.
  - Eye contact
  - Overt behavior and psychomotor activity
  - Attitude
    - Cooperative
    - Hostile
    - Uncooperative

- Distant
- Aloof
- Mode of arrival

2. Mood and affect
   - *Mood:* pervasive or sustained emotion
   - *Affect:* present emotional responsiveness:
     - *Blunted:* severe decrease feeling tone
     - *Restricted:* decreased intensity of feeling tone
     - *Flat:* absence of emotional feeling tone
   - Appropriate versus mood incongruence
   - The psychotic content (hallucinations or delusions) is inconsistent with the prevailing mood.
   - In general, the presence of mood-congruent psychotic features in a mood disorder is indicative of a *poor prognosis.*

3. Speech
   - Quality
   - Rate
   - Spontaneity
   - Rapid and pressured
   - Rambling
   - Hesitant
   - Mumbled
   - Loud

4. Perception
   - Hallucinations
     - Auditory
     - Visual
     - Olfactory
     - Tactile
     - Gustatory
     - Somatic
     - Command

- *Mood-congruent hallucination:* the content is consistent with the client's mood (e.g., depressed, manic). For example, the client in a manic episode hears voices that tell him he is "Paul Revere" or other names that suggest inflated worth.
- *Mood-incongruent hallucination:* the content is inconsistent with the client's mood. For example, the client who is depressed and feels extreme guilt may have hallucinations that centers on themes of inflated self worth.
- Illusions: misinterpretation of external stimuli (e.g., shadow misinterpreted as a ghost)
- Circumstances of hallucinations or illusions (i.e., stress, falling asleep)
- Content

5. Thought processes
   - Loose associations (unrelated, disconnected thoughts)
   - Flight of ideas (rapid thinking, connected and related thoughts)
   - Racing thoughts: rapid thoughts often reflected in rapid and pressured speech. It is one of the hallmark symptoms of manic episode, bipolar I disorder
   - Tangentiality: inability to integrate thoughts resulting in a failure to reach a desired goal
   - Circumstantiality: indirect speech characterized by overinclusion of information with a substantial delay in answering the question

- Clang: association of words similar in sound that includes rhyming
- Blocking: abrupt cessation in train of thought before a thought or idea is completed
- Neologism: new word created by the client
- Perseveration: repetition of words, phrases; persistent response to a previous stimuli

6. Thought content
   - Delusion: a false belief; types:
     - Persecutory (most common)
     - Jealousy
     - Paranoid
     - Somatic
     - Grandiose
   - Preoccupations
   - Obsessions
   - Paranoia
   - Phobias
   - Suicidal/homicidal
   - Ideas of reference
7. Sensorium and cognition
   - Consciousness
   - Orientation
   - Attention
   - Concentration
   - Memory
8. Levels of memory
   - Remote: distant past
   - Recent: last few days
   - Recent past: last few months
   - Immediate retention and recall (seconds to minutes)
   - Reaction to memory loss

9. Higher brain function
   - Visual spatial ability: assess by asking the client to draw the face of a clock or geometric figure.
      - Abstract versus concrete thinking: Proverbs can be used to assess abstract thinking—but they must be familiar to the client. Abstract thinking refers to the ability to use proverbs and metaphors appropriately, such as "raining cats and dogs" refers to torrential rain (abstract) rather than literally cats and dogs falling from the sky (concrete).
   - Concrete thinking is reflected when the client explains a proverb by using the literal meaning of the proverb
   - Information and intelligence
   - Judgment "what if" questions
   - Insight
   - Reliability
E. Suicide Assessment
   - Ask if the client is having thoughts about killing self or others
   - Inquire into static and dynamic risk factors, warning signs, and impact of psychosocial stressors and coping patterns.
   - Thoroughly assess the meaning of client's suicidal plan, including chances of rescue, preparation or rehearsal of suicide plan, and availability of firearms.
   - Inquire about past history of suicide, including precise nature of attempt, number of attempts, reasons for attempt(s), such as psychosocial stressors and life event (crisis).

- Inquire about family history of suicide, including relationship to client, understanding of the attempt or suicide, and response to the incident.

1. High-risk groups
   - European Americans (increases with age)
   - Native Americans (American Indian/Alaskan Native, especially among adolescents)
   - African Americans
   - Hispanic or Latino Americans
   - Asian Pacific Islander Americans

2. High risk factors
   - Psychosocial risk factors (**Table 3-1**)
   - Psychiatric disorders, particularly coexisting psychiatric or medical conditions (**Table 3-2**)
   - Previous history of suicide attempts, gestures, ideations, threats
   - Positive family history (Mann & Currier, 2007; Steele & Doey, 2007)

3. Imminent risk factors
   - Client has a plan (how detailed? means? intent? access to firearms?)
   - Level of lethality
   - Active thoughts of wishes to die and sense of hopelessness and helplessness
   - Obsessive thoughts of dying
   - Poor alliance with staff
   - Command hallucinations that tell the client to kill self
   - Recent trauma or changes in health
   - Force to die is stronger than the wish to live
   - Drug/alcohol intoxication or withdrawal
   - Marked anxiety or panic state (Mann & Currier, 2007)

Table 3-1 Psychosocial Risk Factors for Suicide

- Previous attempt(s)
- Positive family history of suicide, suicide attempts
- Availability of firearms (> 60% of people who kill themselves across the life span use firearms)
- Isolation
- Inadequate or poor social support systems
- Ineffective coping skills
- Hopelessness
- Impulsivity
- Significant stressors, losses, bereavement, and grief
- Emotional turmoil
- Relationship problems, marital turmoil
- Unemployment
- Financial ruin and legal problems
- History of trauma, childhood abuse
- Substance use disorders
- Poor adherence to medication regimen and treatment plan
- Self-destructive behaviors
- Being single
- Shame, humiliation
- Fear of punishment
- Physical illness and declining health and quality of life

- High level of perturbation increases the risk or lethality of suicide
4. Safety of the in-patient
   - Ensure proper hand-off procedures
   - Maintain a safe and therapeutic environment
     - Weight-tested breakaway hardware
     - Protected electrical outlets
     - Windows restricted with maximum opening of 6 inches or locked to protect being opened by the client

Table 3-2   Psychiatric Disorders Relevant to Suicide

Psychiatric Disorder	Prevalence or Risk Factors
Schizophrenia	• 4–9% • Early in course of illness (within 1–6 years of diagnosis) • Later onset of illness • Presence of command hallucinations, marked agitation, depression, sense of inadequacy, intense guilt • Significant depressive symptoms during residual phases • Substance use • White race • Previous attempts • Poor adherence to treatment • Lack of social support
Major depression	• 2–15% • Within the first year of illness and shortly after discharge • Co-occurring anxiety and/or anxiety disorders • Anhedonia or loss of pleasure or interests • Substance use • Cognitive deficits (decreased concentration) • Indecisiveness • Sleep disturbances • Hopelessness • History of previous suicide attempts
Bipolar disorder	• 8–19% • Male gender • Previous suicide attempts • Hopelessness • Substance use disorders, especially alcohol misuse • Poor adherence to medication regimen
Personality disorder, borderline personality disorder	• Impulsivity and aggression interact to increase suicide risk • May be the result of impulsivity, a core feature of the disorder, interacting with violent-aggressive tendencies • Co-existing psychiatric disorder • Childhood trauma, including various forms of abuse

- Ceiling free of hanging objects
- Secured housekeeping carts and closets
- Timely and accurate documentation
- Nonbreakable glass windows or partitions
- One-to-one and environmental surveillance
- Clinical rounds to assess environment of care and potential risk factors
- Bed position
- Daily risk assessment of self-harm or harm to others
- Clear policy for staff orientation and guideline

5. Legal considerations
   - Perform a complete documentation of the suicide attempt/ideations and the decision-making process for discharge
   - Develop a postdischarge and aftercare plan
   - Make appropriate referrals (call and confirm)
   - Provide written instructions to family/client
   - Perform weapons assessment and document findings
   - Instruct family/client to call on interim basis as needed (Antai-Otong, 2004)

F. Psychiatric Rating Scales
   Rating scales serve to standardize the data collected across time and by diverse clinicians. It offers clinicians and clients an opportunity to monitor symptoms in relation to medications and other interventions to determine symptoms management and treatment efficacy. The follow-

ing are examples of various tools used to assess symptoms and treatment response over time.

1. Psychotic symptoms
   - Brief Psychiatric Rating Scale (BPRS)
   - Scale for the Assessment of Negative Symptoms (SANS)
   - Positive and Negative Syndrome Scale (PANSS)
   - Yale Manic Rating Scale (YMRS)
2. Depressive symptoms
   - Beck Depression Inventory (BDI)
   - Hamilton Rating Scale for Depression (HRSD/HAM-D)
   - Geriatric Depression Scale (GDS)
   - Depression SIG E CAPS (mnemonic):
     - **S**leep disturbances
     - **I**nterest (loss of or anhedonia)
     - **G**uilt or sense of worthlessness
     - **E**nergy (decreased)
     - **C**oncentration difficulties
     - **A**ppetite disturbances
     - **P**sychomotor retardation or agitation
     - **S**uicidal thoughts
3. Movement assessment scales
   - Abnormal Involuntary Movement Scale (AIMS)
   - Simpson-Angus Rating Scale for Extrapyramidal Side Effects (Simpson-Angus Scale)
   - Barnes Akathisia Rating Scale (BARS)
4. Anxiety
   - Rating scale for assessing current and lifetime PTSD (CAPS)
   - Clinicians Administered PTSD Scale (CAPS)
   - Hamilton Anxiety Rating Scale (HAM-A)

- Panic Disorder Severity Scale (PDSS)
- Yale-Brown Obsessive Compulsive Scale (YBOCS)
- Zung Self-Rating Anxiety Scale (SAS)

5. Functional status
   - Clinical Global Impression (CGI)
   - Graphic Rating Scale (GRS)
   - Global Assessment of Functioning (GAF) scale
   - The MOS 36-item Short Form Health Survey (SF-36)

6. Cognitive function
   - Mini Mental State Examination (MMSE)

7. Psychiatric diagnoses
   - Structured Clinical Interview for DSM-III-R (SCID)
   - Structured Clinical Interview for DSM-III-R Personality Disorder (SCID II)

8. Substance-related disorders
   - Addiction Severity Scale (ASI)
   - CAGE (mnemonic based on four questions):
     - Have you ever felt the need to **cut** down on drinking?
     - Have people **annoyed** you by criticizing your drinking?
     - Have you ever felt bad or **guilty** about your drinking?
     - Have you ever had a drink first thing in the morning (**eye opener**) to steady your nerves or to get rid of a hangover?
   - Alcohol Use Disorders Identification Test (AUDIT)
   - Clinical Institute Withdrawal Assessment for Alcohol scale (CIWA-Ar)

G. *Diagnostic and Statistical Manual of Mental Disorders,* Fourth Edition, Text Revision *(DSM-*

IV-TR) Classification (American Psychiatric Association, 2000)

- Axis I: Clinical Disorders; other conditions that may be a focus of clinical attention
- Axis II: Personality Disorder; Mental Retardation
- Axis III: General Medical Conditions
- Axis IV: Psychosocial and Environmental Problems
- Axis V: Global Assessment of Functioning (GAF)

■ References

American Psychiatric Association. (2000). *Diagnostic and statistical manual of mental disorders* (4th ed., text revision). Washington, DC: Author.

Antai-Otong, D. (2004). *Psychiatric emergencies.* Eau Claire, WI: Professional Educational Systems, Inc.

Mann, J. J., & Currier, D. (2007). A review of prospective studies of biologic predictors of suicidal behavior in mood disorders. *Archives of Suicide Research, 11,* 3–16.

Steele, M. M., & Doey, T. (2007). Suicidal behaviour in children and adolescents. part 1: Etiology and risk factors. *Canadian Journal of Psychiatry, 52*(Suppl 1), 21S–33S.

Sullivan, J. T., Sykora, K., Schneiderman, J., Naranjo, C. A., & Sellers, E. M. (1989). Assessment of alcohol withdrawal: The revised clinical institute withdrawal assessment for alcohol scale (CIWA-Ar). *British Journal of Addiction, 84,* 1353–1357.

Yesavage, J. A., Brink, T. L., Rose, T. L., Lum, O., Huang, V., Adey, M. B., et al. (1983). Development and validation of a geriatric depression screening scale: A preliminary report. *Journal of Psychiatric Research, 17,* 37–49.

- Safety (lethality in overdose)
- Side effects (long term): sexual disturbances, sedation, agitation, weight gain
- Drug interactions or coexisting medical conditions
- Cost (affordability)
- Neurotransmitter specificity-target site? Serotonergic or adrenergic or both?

2. Bipolar disorder type I (manic, depressed, or mixed episodes): a distinct period of abnormal and persistently elevated, expansive, irritable mood lasting at least *1 week* (APA, 2000)
   - Expansive, elated, or agitated mood
   - Decreased need for sleep
   - Racing thoughts
   - Circumstantial, tangential, and pressured speech
   - Increased involvement with pleasurable activities
   - Intrusiveness
   - Talkativeness
   - A risk of violence toward self and others

3. Bipolar disorder type II (hypomanic, depressed, or mixed episodes)
   - Major depressive episode
   - History of hypomania
   - Mixed

B. Major Psychotic Disorders
   1. Schizophrenia: Refers to a brain disorder and is considered a psychotic condition of multidimensional causes. Persistence of illness for at least 6 months (including prodrome) and persistence of the active phase for at least 4 weeks, consisting of one of the following:
      - Disturbances in behavior, thinking, feeling, and perception

- Bizarre delusions: false beliefs stemming from inaccurate external inference; do not reflect the individual's culture intelligence and cannot be corrected by reasoning or logic
- Hallucinations: distorted perceptions of reality that arise from alterations in complex internal processes; auditory, such as "hearing voices" that others do not hear, or visual, "seeing things" that others do not see
- Disorganized speech
- Disorganized or catatonic behavior
- Negative symptoms (APA, 2000)
- Agitation and irritability
- Restlessness
- Impulsive aggression

Symptoms of schizophrenia are listed as negative, positive, or cognitive.

- *Negative symptoms:* A loss or a decrease in the ability to initiate plans, speak, express feelings, and experience pleasure in activities of daily living. They are target symptoms of atypical antipsychotic medications (Stahl & Buckley, 2007).
- *Positive symptoms:* Manifest as alterations in thoughts or perceptions and include hallucinations, delusions, thought disorder, and disorders of movement.
- *Cognitive symptoms:* Manifest as alterations in working memory (keeping information focused), executive function, semantic memory (verbal fluency), visual memory, and verbal memory; are considered core features of the schizophrenia.

There are 5 major subtypes of schizophrenia:

- Paranoid: characterized by the presence of persecutory delusions or delusions of grandeur
- Undifferentiated: marked delusions, hallucinations, disorganized thoughts and behavior
- Residual: absence of marked delusions, hallucinations, incoherence, or disorganized behavior
- Disorganized: marked by regressive, chaotic, or primitive behavior
- Catatonic: characterized by marked disturbances in motor function called waxy flexibility; stupor; posturing (APA, 2000)

See Table 5-2 for an in-depth discussion of nursing interventions for clients who present with acute symptoms.

2. Schizoaffective disorder: Persistent period during which there is either a major depressive episode or manic episode or a mixed episode that occurs concurrently with symptoms that meet criteria A for schizophrenia (APA, 2000):
   - Delusions
   - Hallucinations
   - Disorganized speech
   - Grossly disorder organized behavior
   - Negative symptoms
3. Delusional disorder: The prominent symptom is non-bizarre delusions. Symptoms do not meet criteria for schizophrenia and function is not markedly impaired. Specific types of delusional disorder include:
   - Erotomanic
   - Grandiose

- Jealousy
- Somatic
- Persecutory (most common type)

4. Treatment: Clients with delusional disorders are highly resistant to treatment, particularly medications, because they hold fast to their delusions and suspiciousness. Each client must be assessed to determine the most appropriate treatment.

5. Substance-induced psychosis and psychosis due to a general medical condition: Discussed later in this book.

C. Anxiety Disorders

1. Panic disorder
   - Manifested as a discrete period of intense fear or discomfort leading to biological manifestations:
     - Palpitations
     - Diaphoresis
     - Shortness of breath
     - Lightheadedness
     - Dizziness
     - Chest discomfort
     - Gastrointestinal distress
     - Derealization
     - Fear of losing control, dying, or going crazy
     - Paresthesias (APA, 2000)
   - High prevalence of coexisting major depression and suicide risk. Evaluate suicide risk throughout treatment.
   - Treatment
     - Mainstay treatment for acute anxiety/panic attacks is benzodiazepines in clients who do not have a history of substance use disorders.

- Maintenance treatment is novel antidepressants, such as selective serotonin reuptake inhibitors and serotonin-norepinephrine reuptake inhibitors (see Table 5-1). (Roy-Byrne et al., 2005)

2. Generalized anxiety disorder
   - Excessive worrying
   - Restlessness
   - Chronic course
   - Muscle tension and trembling
   - Agitation
   - Free-floating anxiety
   - Sleep disturbances (APA, 2000)
   - High co-occurrence with major depression and substance use disorder
   - More common in older adults than other anxiety disorders
   - High suicide rate

3. Obsessive-compulsive disorder
   - *Obsessions:* recurrent persistent thoughts, impulses, or images that produce anxiety and distress
   - *Compulsions:* repetitive behaviors or mental acts performed in response to obsessions (APA, 2000)

4. Posttraumatic stress disorder
   - Exposure to an overwhelming traumatic or stressful event that threatens life, integrity (longer than 4 weeks)
   - Nightmares
   - Flashbacks
   - Autonomic arousal
   - *Intrusive:* repeated reliving of the event
   - *Avoidance:* inability to remember important aspects of the event, feeling de-

tached, avoiding people, places, and objects
  - *Arousal:* irritability, difficulty concentrating, insomnia, hypervigilance, exaggerated startle response (APA, 2000)
5. Social anxiety disorder (SAD)
  - Marked persistent fear of one or more social or performance situations
  - Arousal of anxiety when exposed to these situations
  - Avoidant behaviors
  - Irrational fear of a specific phobia(s) (APA, 2000)
6. Treatment: The treatment of anxiety disorders was previously mentioned under panic disorder. An integrated approach that involves both pharmacological and psychotherapeutic interventions, such as cognitive behavioral therapy, desensitization, and group and family therapy, has demonstrated efficacy in the treatment of anxiety disorders.

D. Substance Use Disorders

Treating the client who presents with a suspected substance use disorder requires a comprehensive physical and mental status examination. It is important to distinguish between substance dependence and substance abuse. According to the APA (2000), *substance dependence* refers to the persistent use of a substance, with or without physical dependence. Physical dependence often manifests after continued use alters physiological homeostasis and cessation results in a specific physiologic syndrome, such as alcohol or opioid withdrawal. In comparison, *substance abuse* refers to maladaptive patterns of consumption that veers from acceptable social norms. Diagnostic studies assist clinicians in making a differential diagnosis and may include:

- Blood alcohol level
- Mean corpuscle volume
- Gamma-glutamyl transferase
- Transaminases (liver enzymes)
- Uric acid
- Triglyceride values
- Toxicology screens
- CAGE or AUDIT (see Section 3)
- Mental status examination
- Complete blood count with differential
- Vitamin B_{12} and folate levels
- Urinalysis
- Renal studies
- Electrocardiogram
- Liver function tests

1. Alcohol
   a. Alcohol intoxication: time limited
      - Smell of alcohol
      - Ataxia
      - Slurred/incoherent speech
      - Nystagmus
      - Blurred vision
      - Coma → death
   b. Alcohol withdrawal
      - Symptoms occur within 4 to 12 hours after cessation or reduction of alcohol consumption:
         - Mild
            - Tremulousness
            - Shakiness
            - Fluctuation in vital signs
            - Anxiety

- Mild gastrointestinal disturbances
- Sleep disturbances (24 to 48 hours)
- Moderate to severe
  - Sensory-perceptual disturbances
  - Severe shakes and tremors
  - Diaphoresis
  - Elevated temperature
  - Nausea/vomiting
  - Fluctuation in vital signs
  - Withdrawal seizures
- Severe withdrawal
  - When left untreated often leads to death, usually occurs after 5 to 15 years of heavy alcohol use
  - Delirium tremens
  - Delirium emerging after cessation of heavy alcohol use (within 48 hours)
  - Profound autonomic hyperactivity: elevated blood pressure, tachycardia, diaphoresis, cardiovascular collapse

c. Acute management
- Administer benzodiazepines to produce sedation and to reduce severity of withdrawal symptoms and risk of seizures
  - Long-acting benzodiazepines
    - *Advantage:* self-tapering secondary to cumulative metabolites
    - *Disadvantage:* cumulative metabolites produce confusion, ataxia, and over-sedation, particularly in older adults or those with compromised liver function

and parenteral absorption is *unpredictable*
- Short-acting benzodiazepines
  - *Advantages:* Parenteral administration is rapid and reliable and fewer cumulative metabolites.
  - *Disadvantage:* Requires frequent dosing, which increases the risk of addiction.

d. Supportive interventions
- Approach in a calm and reassuring manner
- Continuously monitor mental and physical status
- Ensure safety—assess for falls, suicide risk and other potential injuries
- Explain all procedures
- Monitor for seizures and other medical emergencies
- Reassure to reduce anxiety and promote orientation
- Administer fluids when indicated along with vitamins and thiamine, and monitor fluid, nutritional, and electrolyte balance.

e. Indications for hospitalization
- History of severe withdrawal
- Moderate withdrawal in the first 12 to 18 hours
- Persistent confusion
- Chest infiltrate
- Psychosis

2. Opioids
   a. Emergencies
   - Hypotension
   - Decreased heart rate

- Decreased respirations: quality and rate
- Pupil constriction
- Hypothermia
- Within 24 hours morphine is excreted but is detectable for > 48 hours
- *Severe overdose*
  - Pinpoint pupils
  - Comatose, semicomatose
  - Rales, cyanosis
  - Shallow respirations
  - Respiratory depression or apnea leading to anoxia

b. Acute management
  - Initiate life support measures
  - Pharmacological interventions
    - Naloxone (Narcan) 2 mg intravenously, subcutaneously, or intramuscularly and then 2 to 4 mg as needed
    - Absence of respiratory depression: 0.4 to 0.8 mg and if no response give 2 mg and repeat as needed (optimal response within 2 to 3 minutes of intravenous injection and 15 minutes after intramuscular or subcutaneous injection)

c. Withdrawal
  - Yawning
  - Diaphoresis
  - Rhinorrhea
  - Tearing
  - Sleeplessness
  - Dilated pupils
  - Gastrointestinal disturbances
  - "Goose bumps"

- Shakes
- Diarrhea
- Aching all over
- Flu-like symptoms
- Intense anxiety and muscle tension
- Increased blood pressure and heart rate

d. Treatment
- Psychosocial
  - Supportive and nonjudgmental attitude
- Pharmacological
  - Clonidine for autonomic arousal symptoms
    - Side effects: decreased blood pressure and pulse rate, orthostatic hypotension, dizziness, sedation
  - Short-term detoxification with methadone and clonidine

3. Buprenorphine (Buprenex, Suboxone, Subutex)
- Approved by the U.S. Food and Drug Administration in 2002
- Provides a less addictive alternative to methadone maintenance
- Reduces cravings with only mild withdrawal symptoms
- Can be prescribed in the privacy of a doctor's office
- Side effects: dizziness, GI disturbances, sweating, headache, liver problems

a. Stimulant-related emergencies
- Increased heart rate and respirations
- Hyperactivity
- Diaphoresis
- Dilated pupils
- Hypervigilance

- Hemorrhagic stroke
- Psychosis
- Agitation
- Chest pain
- Cardiac arrest
- Violence
- Seizures
- Fever

  b. Treatment
  - Haloperidol + lorazepam (2 to 5 mg intramuscularly or intravenously; short-acting for stimulant-induced psychosis); one to two doses every 30- to 60-minute intervals produces rapid and prolonged sedation
  - Monitor mental and physical status
  - Document response and symptom control

E. Eating Disorders

These are a group of psychiatric disorders marked by significant disturbance in eating behavior. There are three major categories.

  1. Anorexia nervosa
  - Potentially fatal psychiatric condition manifested by disturbed body image and self-imposed dietary limitations that frequently result in significant malnourishment.
  - Clients lack insight into their distorted body image and have a persistent need to be thin by both purging and excessive exercise.
  - Mortality ranges between 5% and 18% of clients.
  - Women are more likely to have an anorexia nervosa.
  - The client has marked fears of gaining

weight or becoming obese although underweight.
- Weight loss is associated with refusal to maintain body weight at or above minimally normal weight for age and height (less than 85% of that expected).
- Specific types include restricting (limited to non-bingeing) and binge eating-purging type (APA, 2000).

a. Treatment
- Long-term hospitalization normally stems from severe malnutrition to restore the client's nutritional state.
- A comprehensive treatment approach is critical to helping the client with an eating disorder.
- Cognitive behavioral, family, and psychopharmacological interventions are the major treatment options for the client with an eating disorder.

2. Bulimia
- Episodic, compulsive, and rapid food consumption of large quantities of food within a short period of time (binge eating) followed by self-induced vomiting, excessive use of laxatives or diuretics, fasting, or excessive exercise
- Two types of bulimia: purging and nonpurging
- Nonpurging bulimia clients have less body image disturbances and are more likely to be overweight

F. Cognitive Disorders
Refers to disorders that result in cognitive disturbances, memory deficits and sleep disturbances. Dementia and delirium are major

cognitive disorders. Dementia is associated with profound cognitive impairment in memory, judgment, intelligence, language, learning attention, and orientation. They are often referred to as reversible and irreversible dementias. Example of reversible dementias or cognitive disturbances include hypothyroidism and decreased folate and B_{12} and normal pressure hydrocephalus. These conditions are often reversed when diagnosed and treated in a timely manner. The most common type of irreversible dementia is Alzheimer's disease.

1. Alzheimer's disease (AD) is the most common irreversible dementia that is characterized by a slow progressive course and characterized by multiple cognitive deficits and behavioral disturbances (APA, 2000). Symptoms emerge over time and often occur in several stages:

    a. Stage I (mild/early)
      - Memory impairment
      - Disorientation
      - Restlessness
      - Anxiety
      - Shortened attention span
      - Impairment in new learning
      - Repeats things over and over again
      - Gets lost easily
      - Lack of interest or initiative
      - Increased suspiciousness, fearfulness

    b. Stage II (moderate)
      - Experiences difficulty with ADLs, such as dressing and self-neglect
      - Exhibits anxiety or depression
      - Exhibits multiple cognitive deficits
      - Believes things are real that are not

- Argues more than usual
- Paces about
- Often requires close supervision

c. Stage III (severe)
- Global cognitive decline
- Loss of personality
- Emotional disinhibition
- Physical impairment
- Inability to use or understand words
- Failure to recognize who they are in mirror

d. Treatment: Although there is no cure for AD, a number of medications are marketed for their usefulness in slowing the progression of this brain disease. Acetylcholinesterase inhibitors are the major medications used to treat various stages of AD (Bottiggi et al., 2007). See Table 5-4 for current medications used to treat AD.

e. Psychosocial interventions: The interventions are guided by the stage of illness. Normally during the moderate and severe stage the nurse must provide a safe and structured environment that promotes self-esteem and respect, provides structure and assistance with activities of daily living, and ensures staff and client safety.
- Explain all procedures
- Keep explanations simple and direct
- Assess self care needs
- Educate the family about AD and refer to community resources for support
- Maintain safe, structured, and caring environment
- Provide structured activities

2. Normal pressure hydrocephalus dementia: Refers to a clinical syndrome that consists of the triad of gait instability associated with frequent falls, incontinence, lack of spontaneity in movement, verbal response and emotionality and decreased ability to process information. These symptoms are coupled with the laboratory findings of normal cerebrospinal fluid (CSF) pressures and radiographic findings of enlarged ventricles. This rare cause of this potentially reversible dementia generally affects persons older than 60 years.

   a. Treatment: The most common treatment is ventriculoperitoneal. This procedure involves the use of general anesthesia (Chaudhry et al., 2007).

3. Delirium: Generally has a rapid and transitory course and often associated with an underlying medical condition that needs to be quickly determined and treated. Major symptoms include:

   - *A rapid onset and are transitory*
   - Disorientation
   - Memory disturbances
   - Easily distracted and hard to engage (attention and concentration disturbances)
   - Lethargy or marked agitation and high potential for violence
   - Perceptual-sensory disturbances, such as visual, tactile, and auditory hallucinations, delusions
   - Emotional disturbances, such as anxiety, fear, depression, euphoria, irritability, anger, and apathy
   - Disturbances in sleep-wake cycle

- Physical: increased heart rate and blood pressure, flushed face, and dilated pupils

Differential diagnosis is critical because it guides in treatment management and clinical outcomes.

    a. Pharmacological interventions
- Administer a low-dose (0.5–5 mg/day) of high-potency antipsychotic, such as haloperidol is useful in treating delusions, paranoia, and perceptual disturbances
- Risperidone 0.5 mg/day increased to 2 mg bid PRN

    b. Psychosocial interventions
- Approach in calm and reassuring manner
- Reduce environmental stimuli
- Keep explanations simple and direct
- Arrange for someone to remain with client at all times
- Assess level of dangerousness
  - Provide adequate lighting
  - Decrease environmental clutter

G. Personality Disorders

These are deeply ingrained maladaptive patterns of thought and behavior that persist across a person's life. Etiology of personality disorders are multidimensional and include childhood trauma, genetic vulnerability, and significant early family turmoil.

1. Major types of personality disorders include three clusters:
- Cluster A: Refers to the odd and eccentric cluster—paranoid, schizoid, and schizotypal personality disorders. Characteristic symptoms include fantasies and projection and a propensity toward psychotic thinking.

- Cluster B: Characterized by dramatic, erratic, and emotional cluster—narcissistic, histrionic, borderline, and antisocial personality disorders.
- Cluster C: Refers to a cluster characterized by anxiety or fearfulness—dependent, avoidant, and obsessive-compulsive personality disorders

2. Borderline personality disorder
   - Affective dysregulation
   - Patterns of chaotic and unstable relationships
   - Intense fears of abandonment
   - Recurrent self-destructive behaviors
   - Low self-esteem
   - Low frustration tolerance
   - Marked identity disturbances
   - Poor boundaries
   - Chronic dysphoria
   - Hypersensitive to object loss
   - Experts at "staff splitting"
   - Pervasive feelings of emptiness
   - Labile affect
   - Intense feelings of anger and rage
   - Demanding, shows contempt for staff
   - Stress-generated brief reactive psychosis (APA, 2000)
   - High concomitance with posttraumatic stress disorder, substance use disorders, and bipolar spectrum disorders
   - Among patients with borderline personality disorder 69% to 80% engage in self-destructive behaviors, such as self-injurious and suicidal behavior (Soloff, Fabio, Kelly, Malone, & Mann, 2005; Soloff, Lynch, Kelly, Malone, & Mann, 2000).

3. Antisocial personality disorder
   - History of childhood conduct disorder or behaviors that parallel diagnostic criteria
   - Disregard for social rules, norms, and cultural codes
   - Impulsive behavior
   - A lack of empathy or regard for the rights and feelings of others
   - A limited range of human emotions
   - Manipulation, exploitation, and violation of the rights of others
   - Often involves criminal behavior
4. Treatment
   - Individuals rarely seek treatment on their own and may only initiate therapy when court ordered.
   - Individuals often lack insight into their behavior or reasons for seeking treatment.
   - Newer treatment such as dialectical behavior therapy has demonstrated efficacy in the treatment of borderline personality disorder because it helps the client cope and modulate stressors and reduce suicidal behaviors (Linehan et al., 2006).

■ References

American Psychiatric Association. (2000). *Diagnostic and statistical manual of mental disorders* (4th ed., text revision). Washington, DC: Author.

Bottiggi, K. A., Salazar, J. C., Yu, L., Caban-Holt, A. M., Ryan, M., & Schmitt, F. A. (2007). Concomitant use of medications with anticholinergic properties and acetylcholinesterase inhibitors: Impact on cognitive and physical functioning in Alzheimer disease. *American Journal of Geriatric Psychiatry, 15,* 357–359.

Chaudhry, P., Kharkar, S., Heidler-Gary, J., Hillis, A. E., Newhart, M., Kleinman, J. T., et al. (2007). Characteristics and reversibility of dementia in Normal Pressure Hydrocephalus. *Behavioural Neurology, 18*, 149–158.

Linehan, M. M., Comtois, K. A., Murray, A. M., Brown, M. Z., Gallop, R. J., Heard, H. L., et al. (2006). Two-year randomized controlled trial and follow-up of dialectical behavior therapy vs therapy by experts for suicidal behaviors and borderline personality disorder. *Archives of General Psychiatry, 63*, 757–766.

Roy-Byrne, P. P., Craske, M. G., Stein, M. B., Sullivan, G., Bystritsky, A., Katon, W., et al. (2005). A randomized effectiveness trial of cognitive-behavioral therapy and medication for primary care panic disorder. *Archives of General Psychiatry, 62*, 290–298.

Soloff, P. H., Fabio, A., Kelly, T. M., Malone, K. M., & Mann, J. J. (2005). High-lethality status in patients with borderline personality disorder. *Journal of Personality Disorders, 19*, 386–399.

Soloff, P. H., Lynch, K. G., Kelly, T. M., Malone, K. M., & Mann, J. J. (2000). Characteristics of suicide attempts of patients with major depressive episode and borderline personality disorder: A comparative study. *American Journal Psychiatry, 157*, 601–608.

Stahl, S. M., & Buckley, P. F. (2007). Negative symptoms of schizophrenia: A problem that will not go away. *Acta Psychiatrica Scandinavia, 115*, 4–11.

each medication's side effect profile, implications for psychoeducation, and symptoms the client and family need to report when they occur. Psychostimulants used to treat attention deficit hyperactivity disorder are associated with the risk of abuse and various gastrointestinal side effects including appetite and weight disturbances (Fawcett, 2005).

Of the adverse side effects associated with antipsychotic medications, neuroleptic malignant syndrome and metabolic syndrome are the most serious and potentially fatal. Metabolic syndrome is associated with atypical antipsychotic medications that cause significant weight gain or obesity namely around the abdomen (increased body mass index), subsequent increased insulin resistance or type 2 diabetes, high triglycerides and low HDL cholesterol, hypertension, and risk of coronary heart disease. Lack of exercise and genetic predisposition are also linked to this serious medical complication (Antai-Otong, 2004). Neuroleptic malignant syndrome is thought to arise from reduced dopamine activity in the brain secondary to dopamine antagonist and reductions of dopamine in the nigrostriatal dopamine neural pathways.

Table 5-1   Pharmacological Interventions

Drug Category	Generic Name (Brand Name)	Dose Range (oral)	Side Effects	Clinical Implications
Antidepressants				
Selective serotonin reuptake inhibitor (SSRI)	Fluoxetine (Prozac)	20–60 mg	GI: nausea (most common) vomiting, diarrhea (esp. sertraline), weight gain	Avoid use of *all ADPs* with MAOIs or within 14 days of discontinuation
	Paroxetine (Paxil)/paroxetine CR	20–60 mg/37.5 (CR)	CV: palpitations, hot flashes	Assess and document symptoms
	Sertraline (Zoloft)	50–200 mg	GU: sexual dysfunction	Obtain baseline physical exam and appropriate lab studies, weight
	Citalopram (Celexa)	20–60 mg	Tremors and akathisia with ↑ dose fluoxetine	Assess for suicide risk throughout treatment and recurrent mania
	Escitalopram (Lexapro)	10–20 mg		Monitor appropriate diagnostic studies, including complete blood count with differential, complete serum chemistries,
	Fluvoxamine (Luvox) (also used in the treatment of OCD)			

continues

			thyroid, liver and renal studies, urinalysis toxicology screens, and VDRL test. Obtain vital signs Health education about side effects, including sexual, GI, and weight gain Instruct to take with meals to reduce GI disturbances
Selective norepinephrine reuptake inhibitor (SNRI)	Venlafaxine, venlafaxine XR (Effexor, Effexor XR)	225 mg/day (divided doses) Venlafaxine XR: 150 mg once/day dosing, up to 225 mg/day	CNS: mania, hypomania, somnolence, dizziness, confusion, depersonalization, paranoia, headaches CV: sustained increased blood pressure, tachycardia, peripheral edema, diaphoresis	Same as SSRIs Monitor blood pressure (SNRIs)
	Duloxetine (Cymbalta)	60–120 mg/day	GI: anorexia, nausea and vomiting, constipation, diarrhea, dry mouth, hemorrhoids, rectal bleeding, mouth ulcer Genitourinary (GU): sexual disturbances	

Table 5-1 Pharmacological Interventions, continued

Drug Category	Generic Name (Brand Name)	Dose Range (oral)	Side Effects	Clinical Implications
Dopamine-norepinephrine reuptake inhibitors	Bupropion (Wellbutrin) (Wellbutrin SR)	200–300 mg/day (bid) 150 (single dose), 400 mg (divided dose)	CNS: somnolence, dizziness, activation of mania/hypomania, sedation, delirium, hallucinations, anxiety, and paranoia ↓ seizure threshold	Note any history of seizures, eating disorders
Norepinephrine-serotonin modulators	Mirtazapine (Remeron)	15–45 mg/day	GI: nausea and vomiting, dry mouth, constipation, ulcer, weight gain, thirst, dehydration, sedation CV: myocardial infarction, hypertension, syncope, migraine, hypotension Hematologic agranulocytosis	Monitor weight, electrocardiogram (ECG), liver and renal function tests

Tricyclic antide-pressants	Clomipramine (Anafranil) (used to treat OCD)	100–250 mg	Cardiotoxic, serious ventricular arrhythmias	Baseline ECG and follow-up ECG
	Nortriptyline (Pamelor)	75–150 mg	Seizures	Health education about oper-ating dangerous machinery
	Imipramine (Tofranil)	150–300 mg	Postural hypotension	Consider taking at bedtime
	Desipramine (Norpramin)	150–300 mg	Sedation	Teach to rise slowly from sitting position
	Amitriptyline (Elavil)	150–300 mg	Anticholinergic properties	
			Urinary retention	
			Weight gain	
			Confusion	
			Delirium	
			Sexual dysfunction	
			GI disturbances	

continues

Table 5-1 Pharmacological Interventions, continued

Drug Category	Generic Name (Brand Name)	Dose Range (oral)	Side Effects	Clinical Implications
Monoamine oxidase inhibitors (MAOIs)	Phenelzine (Nardil)	60–90 mg (divided doses)	Orthostatic hypotension	Provide health dietary restrictions (tyramine-containing foods), and risk of hypertensive crisis
	Tranylcypromine (Parnate)	10–60 mg	Drowsiness, sedation	Avoid aged foods, such as cheeses, Chianti wine, bananas, antidepressant (ADP) medications to avoid drug interactions (e.g., serotonin syndrome)
			Sexual problems	Avoid cold preparations
				Monitor blood pressure for orthostatic hypotension

continues

Antipsychotic Medications

Atypicals	Quetiapine (Seroquel)	300–800 mg	Orthostatic hypotension	Monitor blood pressure
			Syncope (early treatment)	Teach to rise slowly from sitting position
			Cataracts	Order baseline liver function test; monitor during treatment
			Sedation	
			↑ liver enzymes	Baseline metabolic studies, including fasting glucose and fasting lipids, body mass index
			EPS, dystonia, NMS	
				Baseline waist circumference
				Perform and document baseline
				Abnormal Involuntary Movement Scale (AIMS) to assess for early signs of tardive dyskinesia (TD) and continue to: monitor every 6 months

Table 5-1   Pharmacological Interventions, continued

Drug Category	Generic Name (Brand Name)	Dose Range (oral)	Side Effects	Clinical Implications
Atypicals, continued	Clozapine (Clozaril)	150–300 mg (divided doses) (maximum dose 900 mg)	↑ weight gain Agranulocytosis, bone marrow depression Marked sedation Sialorrhea Low incidence of EPS and tardive dyskinesia Anticholinergic effects, postural hypotension ↑ seizure risk	Special guidelines for treatment-refractory clients Baseline metabolic studies, including lipid studies and fasting glucose Perform body mass index Follow FDA protocols that include frequent CBC with differential
	Risperidone (Risperdal)	2–6 mg	EPS, dystonia, NMS, TD ↑ prolactin levels Sexual side effects Menstrual irregularities	Same as above

continues

Drug	Dose	Side Effects	Monitoring
Ziprasidone (Geodon)	80–160 mg divided doses	EPS, dystonia, NMS Low incidence of weight gain Conduction disturbances: QTc prolongation	Same as above Baseline ECG; monitor during treatment
Aripiprazole (Abilify)	15–30 mg (once a day)	EPS, dystonia, NMS Minimal weight gain	Same as above
Olanzapine (Zyprexa)	5–20 mg	↑ weight gain, risk of metabolic syndrome Sedation EPS, dystonia	Same as above
Olanzapine/fluoxetine (Symbyax)	6 mg/25 mg to 12 mg/50 mg	↑ weight gain, risk of metabolic syndrome Sedation EPS, dystonia	Same as above

Table 5-1 Pharmacological Interventions, continued

Drug Category	Generic Name (Brand Name)	Dose Range (oral)	Side Effects	Clinical Implications
Typicals/ conventional	Haloperidol (Haldol)	5–20 mg	EPS, tardive dyskinesia, NMS	Order baseline ECG, serum electrolytes, especially potassium and magnesium and liver function test; monitor during treatment
	Perphenazine (Trilafon)	12–64 mg	Sedation, QT prolongation and torsades de pointes—primarily with off-label IV administration	Assess familial history of QT prolongation
	Trifluoperazine (Stelazine)	2–40 mg	Anticholinergic properties	Baseline metabolic studies; body mass index
			Endocrine disturbances, sexual problems, menstrual irregularities, weight gain	Perform and document baseline (AIMS) and monitor every 6 months

Anxiolytic Antianxiety Agents

Benzodiazepines	Clonazepam (Klonopin)	0.5–4.0 mg	CNS depressant, sedation, ataxia, dependence, teratogenesis	Avoid operating dangerous equipment Monitor for signs of tolerance, abuse, and dependence (e.g., client starts to increase dose) Caution in clients with a history of substance use disorder Avoid using with other CNS depressants
	Alprazolam (Xanax)	0.5–6.0 mg	Same as clonazepam	Same as clonazepam
	Diazepam (Valium)	2.5–40 mg	Same as clonazepam	Same as clonazepam
	Chlordiazepoxide (Librium)	10–100 mg	Same as clonazepam	Same as clonazepam
	Oxazepam (Serax)	15–120 mg	Same as clonazepam	Same as clonazepam
Nonbenzodiazepines	Buspirone (Buspar)	30–60 mg (bid)	Dizziness, headache, light-headedness, nausea	Encourage to take with food

continues

Table 5-1 Pharmacological Interventions, continued

Drug Category	Generic Name (Brand Name)	Dose Range (oral)	Side Effects	Clinical Implications
Antimanic Agents				
Mood stabilizers (anticonvulsants)	Lamotrigine (Lamictal)	50–200 mg	Sedation, teratogenesis, toxic rash, cognitive blunting, weight changes (neutral)	Educate client and family about rash and symptoms to report
				No serum monitoring required
				Obtain baseline labs, including pregnancy test (applicable to all mood stabilizers)
	Oxcarbazepine (Trileptal)	600–1,200 mg/day	Sedation, ataxia, paresthesias, GI disturbances, abdominal pain, muscle weakness, rash, hyponatremia	Teach to avoid other CNS depressants
				Monitor electrolytes
	Tiagabine (Gabitril)	4–56 mg (divided doses)	Sedation, ataxia, paresthesias, GI disturbances, abdominal pain, muscle weakness, ecchymosis	

Drug	Dose	Adverse effects	Interventions
Topiramate (Topamax)	50–400 mg (bid dosing)	Kidney stones, metabolic acidosis, neurotoxic sedations, tremors, weight loss	Encourage fluids and hydration, monitor chemistries Does not require serum monitoring
Valproic acid, valproate (Depakote, Depakene, Divalproex)	750–4,200 mg (divided doses)	Teratogenic, sedation, neurotoxic, weight gain, endocrine disturbances, polycystic ovary (childbearing women), rash, pancreatitis, increased liver enzymes, toxic rash	Therapeutic dose range 50–100 µ/mL Requires serum monitoring Onset of action 10–14 days Baseline liver function tests; monitor during treatment Do not crush enteric-coated tablets
Carbamazepine (Tegretol)	800–1,200 mg (divided doses)	Sedation, neurotoxic agranulocytosis, teratogenic, toxic rash, weight gain, endocrine disturbances	Therapeutic dose: 4–12 µ/mL Requires serum monitoring Onset of action 10–14 days Baseline CBC with differential; monitor for aplastic anemia; educate family about persistent sore throat and cold (report to provider)

continues

Table 5-1 Pharmacological Interventions , continued

Drug Category	Generic Name (Brand Name)	Dose Range (oral)	Side Effects	Clinical Implications
Lithium	Lithobid, Eskalith	600–1,800 mg	Hypothyroidism, neurotoxic, sedation, ataxia, weight gain, sexual side effects, hormonal changes, nephrotoxic, alopecia, rash	0.6–1.2 mEq/L (acute) Requires serum monitoring Onset of action 10–14 days Baseline thyroid function test, blood urea nitrogen, renal studies; monitor throughout treatment
Attention Deficit Hyperactivity Disorder Agents				
Psychostimulants	Atomoxetine (Strattera)	40–100 mg	Applicable to all psychostimulants, except where noted Anorexia, nauseas, weight loss Insomnia, nightmares Dizziness Rebound phenomena	Baseline weight, height, blood pressure, monitor throughout treatment Baseline diagnostic lab studies; liver function test (monitor)

Section 5 Interventions 71

		Irritability Dysphoria, moodiness, agitation Drug interactions Hepatitis/liver injury (atomoxetine) Dependency	
Dextroamphetamine + amphetamine (Adderall)	5–40 mg	Same as atomoxetine (except liver injury)	Baseline weight, height, blood pressure, monitor throughout treatment Baseline diagnostic lab studies
Methylphenidate (Ritalin)	10–40 mg	Same as atomoxetine (except liver injury)	Same as above
Methylphenidate HCL (Concerta)	18–54 mg	Same as atomoxetine (except liver injury)	Same as above

Antidepressant (ADP); bid, twice daily; CBC, complete blood count; CNS, central nervous system; CV, cardiovascular; ECG, electrocardiogram; EPS, extrapyramidal symptoms; FDA, U.S. Food and Drug Administration; GI, gastrointestinal; GU, genitourinary; NMS, neuroleptic malignant syndrome; OCD, obsessive-compulsive disorder.

Table 5-2   Nursing Interventions for the Client with Acute Psychosis

Major nursing goals:

- *Approach* the client cautiously and respectfully.
- *Convey* confidence, empathy, and concern.
- *Talk* to the client. Call the client by name; introduce yourself but maintain a safe distance in order to reduce anxiety and prevent worsening symptoms.
- *Provide* simple explanations about your concerns and your goal of helping the client.
- *Rule out* delirium, intoxication, or other medical conditions; determine if symptoms are primarily a result of a psychotic disorder.
- *Triage.* Identify serious medical problems (attempt to take vital signs and perform a focused exam). It is imperative to evaluate and rule out medical conditions as the basis of the client's symptoms.
- *Manage* symptoms of arousal with sedation to mitigate anxiety, agitation, and psychotic symptoms.
- *Administer* parenteral antipsychotics and benzodiazapines, such as lorazepam to achieve a maximum concentration.
- *Contain* violence.
- *Recognize* that most clients perceive involuntary medication as traumatic. Explain all procedures and reassure the client that you want to help.
- Call the client by name.
- Avoid approaching an overtly hostile, aggressive client alone.
- Maintain a safe distance, at least leg's length, and avoid invading the client's personal space
- Avoid touching the client or making sudden movements.
- Be cognizant of personal feelings/reactions and maintain a calm demeanor.
- Decrease environmental stimuli.
- Assess the presence and nature of the client's hallucinations or delusions.
- Help the client focus on things in the environment.
- Avoid arguing with the client or discounting the presence of hallucinations, illusions or delusions.
- Assess the client's level of dangerousness, which includes past history of violence towards self or others.

Section 5 Interventions   73

continues

Table 5-3 Antipsychotic Agents: Adverse Drug Reactions and Side Effects

Drug-Induced Adverse Side Effects	Onset of Symptoms	Signs and Symptoms	Treatment and Interventions
Acute dystonia	10% of all clients experience this disorder Usually within hours to days of treatment Most common with intramuscular doses and high potency agents, such as haloperidol	Intense involuntary spasms of muscles of the trunk, tongue, face, jaw, or eyes Abnormal posturing of neck, trunk, and head Impaired swallowing Thick tongue producing slurred speech Eye deviation upward and lateral movement	Immediate intervention Reassure client and educate about symptoms Prophylaxis treatment Intramuscular anticholinergic agents (e.g., 1–2 mg benztropine or 25–50 mg diphenhydramine) Decrease dose or change medication Monitor side effects from anticholinergic agents
Akathisia	Higher incidence in middle-aged women at highest risk Likely to occur during early treatment (within 4 weeks of increasing or initiating high dosages and high potency agents)	Subjective restlessness compared with observation Fidgeting Rocking from one foot to another Sense of anxiety, agitation Pacing	Administer anticholinergic agents; propranolol (Inderal) 30–120 mg/day Benzodiazepine acute and severe agitation and anxiety Consider changing medication

Table 5-3	Antipsychotic Agents: Adverse Drug Reactions and Side Effects, continued		
Drug-Induced Adverse Side Effects	Onset of Symptoms	Signs and Symptoms	Treatment and Interventions
Parkinsonism	10% among those taking antipsychotics (usually within 5–90 days of initiation) Women are twice as likely to experience than men after age 40 50% require continued treatment because symptoms may persist 2 weeks after treatment	Muscle stiffness Shuffling gait Drooling Coarse tremor Blunted facial expressions	Anticholinergic agents
Tardive dyskinesia (TD)	Higher incidence in women No known cure 5% incidence in young adults and 30% after 1 year of treatment in older adults	Involuntary, dyskinetic movement Early symptoms: THINK FACE Tongue, movement, grimacing, blinking, and frowning	Early detection through regular examinations: at least every 6 months is recommended by the APA TD Task Force

Neuroleptic malignant syndrome (NMS)	Onset can occur within a week of exposure to an oral antipsychotic agent and 1 month after exposure to a depot antipsychotic agent	Hyperthermia ($> 38°C$)	Important to make an accurate diagnosis that is usually based on history of exposure to antipsychotic medication
		Severe muscle rigidity	
		Diaphoresis	*Emergency interventions:*
		Dysphagia	Stop all psychotropics!
	Risk factors	Elevated or labile blood pressure	Initiate life support measures
	Dehydration	Incontinence	Increase oxygen
	Mood disorders	Mental status changes, ranging from confusion to coma	Reduce temperature
	Systemic infections, dehydration	Renal failure $2°$ or secondary to myoglobinuria	Stabilize blood pressure and heart rate
	Neurologic conditions, including mental retardation	Tachycardia	Monitor vital signs
	Concurrent lithium treatment	Leukocytosis (elevated white blood cell count)	Hydrate!
	High potency antipsychotics, such as haloperidol	Lab evidence of muscle injury (i.e., elevated creatine phosphokinase)	Administer muscle relaxant: dantrolene (Dantrium); bromocriptine (Parlodel) 20–30 mg/day in four divided doses
	Psychotic agitation	Tremor	
	Previous history of NMS		Treatment usually takes 5–10 days
	Mortality rate 10–30%		

Table 5-4 Common Medications Used to Treat Alzheimer's Disease (Cholinesterase Inhibitors)

Name	Dose (Oral)	Side Effects	Nursing Interventions
Donepezil	5 mg/day	GI disturbances	Dosing: start low and go slow
			Use with caution or avoid use with nonsteroidal anti-inflammatory inhibitor drugs (NSAIDs) (e.g., ibuprofen or aspirin) to prevent stomach ulcers and irritation
			Monitor weight (baseline)
			Provide patient and family health education about side effects to report, such as persistent vomiting or diarrhea
Rivastigmine	1.5 mg twice/day	GI disturbances, weight loss, muscle weakness; rare side effect is gastrointestinal bleeding	Same as above
Galantamine	4 mg twice/day	GI disturbances, weight loss	Same as above
Memantine	5 mg/day	Dizziness, headache, constipation, cognitive disturbances, skin rash, high blood pressure	Same as above, plus: Assess and monitor fall risk Monitor blood pressure

* Major side effects are associated with higher doses.

References

Antai-Otong, D. (2004). Metabolic effects associated with atypical antipsychotic medications. *Perspectives in Psychiatric Care, 40,* 70–72.

Fawcett, J. (2005). Sympathomimetics and dopamine receptor agonists. In B. J. Sadock & V. A. Sadock (Eds.), *Kaplan & Sadock's comprehensive textbook of psychiatry* (8th ed., pp. 2938–2943). Philadelphia: Lippincott Williams & Wilkins.

Marder, S. R., & Van Kammen, D. P. (2005). Dopamine receptor agonists (typical antipsychotics). In B. J. Sadock & V. A. Sadock (Eds.), *Kaplan & Sadock's comprehensive textbook of psychiatry* (8th ed., pp. 2817–2838). Philadelphia: Lippincott Williams & Wilkins.

Takeda, A., Loveman, E., Clegg, A., Kirby, J., Picot, J., Payne, E., et al. (2006). A systematic review of the clinical effectiveness of donepezil, rivastigmine, and galantamine on cognition, quality of life, and adverse events in Alzheimer's disease. *International Journal of Geriatric Psychiatry, 21,* 17–28.

Van Kammen, D. P., & Marder, S. R. (2005). Serotonin-dopamine antagonists (atypical or second-generations antipsychotics). In B. J. Sadock & V. A. Sadock (Eds.), *Kaplan & Sadock's comprehensive textbook of psychiatry* (8th ed., pp. 2914–2938). Philadelphia: Lippincott Williams & Wilkins.

Documentation of these situations must include precisely what the client stated; violence-risk assessment; history of threat and violence; and interventions, such as informing the police or detaining the client.

All states require clinicians to immediately report suspected child or elderly abuse. Confidentiality is limited to the potential or actual harm to these populations.

Ethical considerations often interface with legal issues and must be an integral part of nurse–client relationships. Ethics in mental health refer to principles of conduct that govern the behavior of nurses and other clinicians. One particular legal and ethical consideration involves boundaries. *Boundaries* define the expected and accepted psychological and social distance between the nurse and the client. An example is the client that asks the nurse for a date or other inappropriate social activities (Antai-Otong, 2006). Maintaining clear boundaries is critical in all client situations, but especially important when working with clients with personality disorders, including borderline and antisocial personality disorders. These clients are experts at limit-testing and require firm and consistent limit-setting as part of their treatment. Examples of boundary issues are self-disclosure and engaging in inappropriate social contact with any client. Although self-disclosure has some therapeutic value, it is based on the nature of the nurse–client relationship, the nurse's comfort level about sharing personal information with the client, and the appropriateness of the clinical situation. Excessive self-disclosure interferes with the therapeutic process, whereas too little interferes with trust and makes it difficult for the client to share pertinent information. *Self-disclosure* is a natural part of nurse–client relationships and includes the nurse's name, educational preparation, and pictures of one's family and children and diplomas. Inappropriate self-disclosure includes sharing personal information about one's family, medical conditions, or other problems. It is critical for the nurse to focus on the client's complaints, convey concern, maintain clear boundaries, and collaborate with the client to establish treatment goals (Antai-Otong, 2006).

Other legal and ethical issues include the right to treatment, the right to refuse treatment, consent of minors, seclusion and restraint, competence, and involuntary hospitalization (Barloon & Hendricks, 2008):

- The right to standard quality of treatment: a fundamental right of every client
- The right to refuse treatment: when the individual is deemed competent and poses no threat to self or others
- Right to the least restrictive environment: States are mandated to provide the least restrictive environments as soon as possible.
- Consent of minors: This definition varies among states and refers to the legal definition of minor and competence to make legal decisions.
- Seclusion and restraint: *Seclusion* is defined as physically confining a client to an area such as placing a client in a locked seclusion room. *Restraint* refers to restriction of movement of the client's limbs, head, or body by the use of a mechanical device such as leather belts. An order is required before using these interventions, which should never be a standing or PRN order. In general, nurses must follow Joint Commission standards that govern the applying, monitoring and removing seclusion and restraints (Joint Commission, 2005).

Parameters for the application of restraints and seclusion include:

- Justification in writing
- Use is restricted to emergency situations to ensure the client's physical safety and only when less restrictive alternatives have been deemed ineffective (e.g., deescalation techniques)
- Application must never be used as punishment or for the convenience of staff
- Employment must be consistent with the client's rights (Joint Commission, 2005)
- Competence refers to one's ability to perform certain functions for a particular legal purpose, such as making a will or managing one's financial affairs

Involuntary hospitalization or commitment is generally necessary when the client poses a threat to self or others or has poor judgment and unable to care for self. Most states allow clinicians to hospitalize clients primarily to provide safety, to allow further observation and evaluation, and to administer treatment to mitigate symptoms and prevent harm.

In summary, nurses must be cognizant of federal and state regulations, laws, and mandates that govern their practice. This brief overview provides some guidance in understanding legal and ethical considerations needed to ensure the client's rights and to promote quality and safe psychiatric nursing care.

▌References

Antai-Otong, D. (2006). Psychiatric patients and ethical issues. In V. D. Lachman (Ed.), *Applied Ethics in Nursing* (pp. 133–144). New York: Springer Publishing Company.

Appelbaum, P. S. (2002). Privacy in psychiatric treatment: Threats and responses. *American Journal of Psychiatry, 159,* 1809–1818.

Barloon, L. F., & Hendricks, A. L. (2008). Legal and ethical con-
    siderations. In D. Antai-Otong (Ed.), *Psychiatric nursing:
    Biological and behavioral concepts* (2nd ed., pp. 194–222).
    Clifton Park, NY: Delmar Cengage Learning.
Joint Commission. (2005). *Restraints and seclusion: Frequently
    asked questions.* Retrieved January 18, 2008, from
    http://www.jointcommission.org/AccreditationPrograms/
    BehavioralHealthCare/Standards/FAQs/Provision+of
    +Care+Treatment+and+Services/Restraint+and
    +Seclusion/Restraint_Seclusion.htm
Leeman, C. P. (2004). Confidentiality and the duty to warn of
    possible harm. Letter to editor. *American Journal of
    Psychiatry, 161,* 583.
Tarasoff v. Regents of the University of California, 13 Cal.3d
    177, 118 Cal. Rptr. 129, 529 P.2d 553 (Cal. 1976).

Table 7-1 Managing Acute Psychosis

Target Symptoms

Disturbances in behavior, thinking, feeling, and perception such as:

- Delusions
- Hallucinations
- Agitation and irritability
- Restlessness
- Impulsive aggression

Goals during Emergency Management

- *Dialogue with* the client and significant others
- *Offer* assistance
- *Triage.* Identify serious medical problems (attempt to take vital signs, focused physical exam, brief visual exam)
- *Rule out* delirium, intoxication, or other medical conditions; determine if symptoms are primary psychotic disorder
- *Manage* symptoms of arousal and agitation with sedation
- *Use* parenteral antipsychotic medications and benzodiazepines, such as lorazepam, to achieve rapid and maximum concentration
- *Anticipate and contain* violence
- *Ensure* patient and staff safety
- *Recognize* that most clients view involuntary medication as traumatic

Pharmacological Interventions

- The client's ability to participate regarding medication is important.
- *Psychiatrists may consider administering despite objection* in a client who is dangerous with acute psychosis.
- Before administering medications, obtain a history regarding
  - Drug allergies
  - History of adverse drug reactions such as neuroleptic malignant syndrome
  - Underlying medical conditions

continues

Table 7-1 Managing Acute Psychosis, continued

- Substance use, including last consumption and withdrawal seizures
- Offer oral medications first when appropriate, otherwise administer
  - Haloperidol 5 mg + 2 mg lorazepam IM every 30-60 min prn
  - Lorazepam 1–2 mg IM or po; repeat × 2 every 45 min
  - Risperidone 2 mg concentrate and 2 mg lorazepam orally
- Consider anticholinergic side effects (i.e., older adults, brain damaged, prior adverse drug reaction)

Psychotherapeutic Interventions

- Treat the client with respect
- Introduce yourself
- Call the client by name
- Do not approach an openly hostile aggressive client alone
- Avoid invading personal space
- Avoid touching or making sudden movements
- Be aware of personal feelings/reactions
- Decrease environmental stimuli
- Assess the nature of hallucinations or delusions
- Help the client focus on things in the environment
- Avoid arguing with the client
- Assess the client's level of dangerousness
- Offer choices when possible to increase the client's sense of control
- Offer food, beverages, blankets, or other comfort measures that do not compromise safety; avoid hot coffee or other beverages
- Inform the client of what is going on
- Enlist family in the evaluation and treatment process

Indications for Hospitalization

- Client poses threat to self or others
- Unstable medical or psychiatric condition

continues

Table 7-1 Managing Acute Psychosis, continued

- Inability to manage self-care needs
- Voluntary versus involuntary

Stable Phase

- Adequate therapeutic response with minimal side effects or toxicity to medication regimen
- Adjust medication dose based on efficacy and tolerability (minimum dose to achieve efficacy)
- Supportive environment with less directive and structure
- Family involvement throughout treatment

Stable Phase: Treatment Goals

- Sustain symptom remission or control
- Monitor for movement disorders
- Mitigate risk and consequences of relapse
- Optimize functioning
- Facilitate process of recovery

Psychosocial Interventions

Individualized to meet client preferences, wishes, cultural, spiritual, and gender needs:

- Psychoeducation individual and family group approaches
- Assertive community treatment
- Social skills training
- Cognitive therapy: key domains
- Understanding between patient and therapist
- Identification of target symptoms; development of individualized cognitive and behavioral strategies to cope with symptoms

Monitoring Patients with Schizophrenia: Movement Disorder

- Monitor clients for extrapyramidal symptoms weekly during acute treatment and until medication dose is stabilized for at least 2 weeks
- Monitor for tardive dyskinesia (baseline) and every 6 months for conventional (first-generation) and every 12 months for atypical (second-generation) antipsychotics

Table 7-2   Cognitive Neurological-Related Emergencies

Condition	Clinical Symptoms	Interventions
Delirium		
Delirium refers to a medical condition that arises from multidimensional factors, including medical conditions and substance use (illicit and licit). Persistent delirium at hospital discharge is associated with chronic cognitive and functional outcomes. Risk factors: • Use of restraints • Malnutrition • Use of bladder catheter • Use of more than three medications	• Disturbances of consciousness, attention, cognition, and perception • Memory deficits, disorientation, language disturbances • Dysarthria: speech and language disturbances • Perceptual disturbances: illusions, hallucinations, misinterpretations • Psychomotor agitation • Alterations in neurological function • Nystagmus • Ataxia Prodromal symptoms may include restlessness, irritability, agitation, distractability, and anxiety (1–3 days before clinical symptoms occur).	• Evaluate and determine underlying cause (differential diagnosis) (generally a reversible condition) • History of symptoms • Vital and neurological signs • Review of current medications, including over-the-counter and herbal preparations • Synthesize data from diagnostic laboratory and other studies • Serum chemistries, electrolytes, thyroid panel, liver and renal studies, alanine and aspartate aminotransferases, complete blood count with differential, chest x-ray, electrocardiogram, arterial blood gases, vitamin B_{12} and folate levels, toxicology screens, VDRL, etc.

Course: Develops over a short period of time (usually hours to days) and is transitory during the course of the day.

Potential outcomes: Stupor, coma, seizures, or death, primarily when undiagnosed and untreated.

When delirium occurs in clients who are medically ill, especially older adults, there is a high mortality rate.

Major causes: Underlying medical conditions; substance intoxication or withdrawal or multiple causes.

Clinical presentation: mental status examination

Treat underlying medical conditions

Pharmacological interventions: Administer antipsychotic medications, such as haloperidol, to manage agitation and psychosis. Haloperidol has anticholinergic side effects and produces relatively less sedation and hypotension.

Psychosocial interventions: Use simple direct language

Reorient as needed

Explain all procedures

Ensure safety—don't leave alone

Reduce noise and avoid excessive stimuli

Ensure adequate lighting

Educate client and family about nature of delirium; encourage family to spend time with client to make feel secure

Anticipate anxiety and respond appropriately

Assist with self-care needs

continues

Table 7-2 Cognitive Neurological-Related Emergencies, continued

Condition	Clinical Symptoms	Interventions
Alzheimer's Disease		
Dementia refers to a degenerative brain condition that is evidence from history, physical exam, or lab findings that disturbance is directly related to physiological consequences of a general medical condition. Types: • HIV disease (irreversible) • Alzheimer's disease (irreversible) • Hypothyroidism (reversible with appropriate treatment) • Vitamin B$_{12}$ deficiency (reversible with appropriate treatment) Alzheimer's disease is an irreversible type of dementia Course: insidious and progressive	Three stages of progressive decline associated with Alzheimer's disease: **Stage I: Mild** • Memory impairment • Disorientation • Restlessness • Anxiety • Shortened attention span • Impairment in new learning • Repeat things over and over again • Get lost easily • Lose interest or initiative • Have difficulty finding names • Lose things	MMSE may provide early evidence of cognitive deficits along with self-reported and family history of memory difficulties. MSE and neuropsychiatric testing provide invaluable information about cognitive and memory disturbances. A provisional diagnosis of Alzheimer's disease is based on a comprehensive physical examination that includes routine and special diagnostic studies, including magnetic resonance imaging or computed tomography to evaluate degenerative brain regions and determine if and when pharmacological agents should be considered to delay the progression of the disease (see Table 5-4).

- Undergo personality change (e.g., suspicious, fearful)

Stage II: Moderate

- Confusion
- Poor or impaired judgment
- Neurological deficits
  - Agnosia
  - Aphasia
  - Apraxia
  - Anomia
- Experience difficulty with activities of daily living, such as dressing and self-neglect
- Exhibit anxiety or depression

Mild to moderate symptoms may be treated with anticholinesterase inhibitors, such as donepezil and rivastigmine.

Behavioral and pharmacological interventions may be used during the late stages of the illness.

Suspiciousness, paranoia, delusions:

- Environmental
  - Well lit
  - Moderate stimulation
  - Familiar objects in view
- Pharmacological
  - Low-dose antipsychotic agent

continues

Table 7-2 Cognitive Neurological-Related Emergencies, continued

Condition	Clinical Symptoms	Interventions
	• Believe things are real that are not	Yelling, shouting, cursing:
	• Argue more than usual	• Environmental
	• Pace about	• Assess for pain
	• Often require close supervision	• Use touch and music therapy
	Stage III: Severe	• Environmental stimuli
	• Global cognitive decline	• Pharmacological
	• Intellectual impairments	• Trazodone, buspirone
	• Loss of personality	Family and caregiver resources:
	• Emotional disinhibition	• The Alzheimer's Association: www.alz.org
	• Physical impairment	• The National Family Caregiver Association: www.nfcacares.org
	• Inability to use or understand words	
	• Failure to recognize who they are in mirror	

Verbal Deescalation

This technique reduces escalation and requires verbal and nonverbal communication skills to reduce anxiety and fears. It also entails understanding how we react to our clients when they are stressed and role modeling assertive behaviors, such as:

- Employing active listening skills
- Using reflective statements
- Focusing
- Giving information
- Seeking clarification
- Presenting reality
- Seeking consensual validation

Tables 7-3 and **7-4** present ways to identify and manage stress and strategies to use when interacting with people in distress.

Self-Mutilation

Self-mutilation is the deliberate alteration or destruction of one's own body tissue without the conscious intent of suicide. It is characterized by low lethality and is sporadic or repetitive. The categories are:

- Major
- Stereotypical
- Superficial/moderate (most common form)

The high-risk groups are persons with:

- Eating disorders
- Substance abuse (acute intoxication)
- Schizoid personality
- Psychosis (e.g., religious and sexual preoccupation, command hallucinations)
- Pervasive developmental disorder (autism)
- Developmental disorders
- Borderline personality disorder

Table 7-3   Impact of Stress on Perceptions and Risk of Violence

Normal Stress

- Provides a keen perceptual field
- Enables one to take in all environment and process information

Moderate Stress

- Perceptual stress field narrows
- Focus on here and now
- Not taking in as much information

Verbal Deescalation

- Use astute observational and active listening skills
- Keep it simple (use direct and short statements)
- Use nonthreatening body language
- Use eye contact
- Speak in normal tone of voice
- Avoid touching or making sudden movements
- Encourage verbalization
- Identify the problem
- Provide reassurance
- Focus on problem solving
- Provide alternatives
- Maintain nonthreatening body language
- Encourage expression of feelings
- Enforce consequences
- Seek to maintain dignity

Severe Stress

- Perceptual field limited
- Client can only focus on one thing
- Processing of information severely limited
- Observe for continued escalation, pacing, restlessness, shouting, threatening gestures
- Implement personal safety skills
- Ensure yourself a quick exit
- Immediately call for help when needed
- Provide therapeutic containment

Table 7-4   Strategies for Talking to Angry People

- Stand on nondominant side
- Use nonthreatening body language
- Avoid glaring eye contact
- Avoid pointing at or touching angry people
- Avoid making sudden movements
- Give information in terms of suggestion rather than instruction
- Ensure that a mechanism to muster help is available

Self-Assessment During Intense Confrontations or Interactions

- How am I reacting?
- How's my tone of voice?
- How's my body language?
- Check personal space
- Am I wearing anything dangerous?
- Pay attention to "gut" feelings

Appraise Behaviors that Indicate Escalation

- Pacing and restlessness
- Uncooperative
- Loud and boisterous speech
- Verbal threats and gestures

Assess the Client

- Fearful or anxious demeanor
- Agitated, angry, or irritable mood
- Stressed or threatened appearance
- Suspicious or hostile behavior
- Any change in behavior
- General physical appearance, including personal grooming,
  hygiene, odor, intoxication
- Claims of mistreatment
- Blames others for problems
- Significant dates
- Cultural/generational uniqueness

Of this list, it occurs most often in clients with borderline personality disorder.

People who self-mutilate carry a lifetime suicide rate of 5% to 10%, and approximately 55% to 85% of self-mutilators have made at least one suicide attempt. These clients tend to:

- Be more depressed, anxious, and impulsive
- Often underestimate the lethality of the act
- Be at a greater risk of suicidal behavior
- Report a history of childhood abuse
- Express chronic urges to hurt self

Suicide in people who self-mutilate is characterized by a sense of rising tension before the act and a preoccupation with strong and persistent urges to harm oneself. A major goal is to control impulsivity. The following pharmacological interventions are used (Allen et al., 2005; Barzman et al., 2005; Perrella, Carrus, Costa, & Schifano, 2007):

- Mood stabilizers and anticonvulsant agents, such as valproic acid, lithium and topiramate
- Antipsychotics
- Tricyclic antidepressants
- Selective serotonin reuptake inhibitors

References

Allen, M. H., Currier, G. W., Carpenter, D., Ross, R. W., Docherty, J. P., Expert Consensus Panel for Behavioral Emergencies 2005. (2005). The expert consensus guideline series. Treatment of behavioral emergencies. *Journal of Psychiatric Practice, 11*(Suppl), 1–5.

Barzman, D. H., DelBello, M. P., Kowatch, R. A., Warner, J., Rofey, D., Stanford, K., et al. (2005). Adjunctive topiramate in hospitalized pediatric patients with bipolar disorders. *Journal of Child Adolescent Psychopharmacology, 15*, 931–937.

Perrella, C., Carrus, D., Costa, E., & Schifano, F. (2007). Quetiapine for the treatment of borderline personality disorder; an open-label study. *Progress in Neuropsychopharmacology in Biological Psychiatry, 31*, 158–163.

- Shoulds, musts
- *Catastrophizing*

Example of how negative or distorted thoughts generate negative feelings, avoidant behaviors and physical symptoms:

Situation (Opportunity for a job promotion)
↓
Negative thoughts (I will never get that promotion; If I don't get that promotion, I will be a failure)
↓
Feelings (Intense anxiety, depressed mood)
↓
Behaviors (Avoids situation and does not seek promotion)
↓
Physical symptoms (Fatigue, sleep, concentration and appetite disturbances)

Nursing Interventions

Cognitive Distortion	Example	Nursing Intervention
All or none thinking	I will never get that promotion. If I don't get that job I will be a failure.	Ask the client to list evidence of supporting data concerning his fears of not getting the job and how that makes him a failure

- *Exposure therapy or systematic desensitization:* These techniques involve gradual exposure to a situation that normally generates intense anxiety. It has been demonstrated to relieve intense fears and anxiety seen in the client with posttraumatic stress disorder who is fearful of a recurrent traumatic event.

- *Progressive desensitization:* This technique requires advanced or graduate training in progressive relaxation and formation of hierarchies of fearful situations.
- *Psychoeducation:* This is an integral part of psychiatric care and is based on the assessment of the client's and family's educational needs or knowledge deficits about psychiatric disorders, medications, relapse prevention, and other strategies to manage and cope with a psychiatric disorder and facilitate recovery.
- *Cognitive behavioral social skills training:* Is a cognitive problem solving approach that is used to help clients who lack important skills necessary to interact with others effectively. It affords the client with schizophrenia opportunities to strengthen problem solving, functional and coping skills and compensatory aids for cognitive deficits (Granholm et al., 2005; Granholm et al., 2007).
- *Stress management:* This technique teaches the client how to control thoughts and physiological responses associated with anxiety and tension. Deep breathing exercises, journaling, exercising and imagery are examples of stress management techniques (Antai-Otong, 2001).

▌References

Antai-Otong, D. (2001). Creative stress-management techniques for self-renewal. *Dermatology Nursing, 13,* 31–32, 35–39.

Antai-Otong, D. (2008). Individual psychotherapy. In D. Antai-Otong (Ed.), *Psychiatric Nursing: Biological and Behavioral Concepts* (pp. 789–811). Clifton Park, NY: Delmar Thomson Learning.

Beck, A. T. (1979). *Cognitive therapy and the emotional disorders.* New York: International Universities Press.